RECIPE JOURNAL

This journal belongs to ______________________________

STUDIO
AIZ

HELLO!

We hope you love your new Recipe Journal!
This journal has been thoughtfully designed to help you capture (and never forget!) your favourite recipes.

Whether you are a skilled and 'seasoned' cook or a new recruit in the kitchen, this book of home recipes is the perfect cooking companion to keep on hand.

Fill these pages with your family favourites or scribble down a new recipe from a friend that you'd like to try.
Create your own recipes or cut and stick recipe inspiration from books and magazines!
Dinner party dishes,
lunchbox ideas,
hearty soups,
secret recipes,
decadent desserts,
or simple 10-minute meals.

We hope your Recipe Journal pages overflow with a collection of recipes just perfect for YOU!

Bon Appétit!

RECIPE:

INGREDIENTS

DIRECTIONS

Notes

RECIPE:

INGREDIENTS

DIRECTIONS

Notes

RECIPE:

INGREDIENTS

DIRECTIONS

Notes

RECIPE:

INGREDIENTS

DIRECTIONS

Notes

RECIPE:

INGREDIENTS

DIRECTIONS

Notes

RECIPE:

INGREDIENTS

DIRECTIONS

Notes

RECIPE:

INGREDIENTS

DIRECTIONS

Notes

RECIPE:

INGREDIENTS

DIRECTIONS

Notes

RECIPE:

INGREDIENTS

DIRECTIONS

Notes

RECIPE:

INGREDIENTS

DIRECTIONS

Notes

RECIPE:

INGREDIENTS

DIRECTIONS

Notes

RECIPE:

INGREDIENTS

DIRECTIONS

Notes

RECIPE:

INGREDIENTS

DIRECTIONS

Notes

RECIPE:

INGREDIENTS

DIRECTIONS

Notes

RECIPE:

INGREDIENTS

DIRECTIONS

Notes

RECIPE:

INGREDIENTS

DIRECTIONS

Notes

RECIPE:

INGREDIENTS

DIRECTIONS

Notes

RECIPE:

INGREDIENTS

DIRECTIONS

Notes

RECIPE:

INGREDIENTS

DIRECTIONS

Notes

RECIPE:

INGREDIENTS

DIRECTIONS

Notes

RECIPE:

INGREDIENTS

DIRECTIONS

Notes

RECIPE:

INGREDIENTS

DIRECTIONS

Notes

RECIPE:

INGREDIENTS

DIRECTIONS

Notes

RECIPE:

INGREDIENTS

DIRECTIONS

Notes

RECIPE:

INGREDIENTS

DIRECTIONS

Notes

RECIPE:

INGREDIENTS

DIRECTIONS

Notes

RECIPE:

INGREDIENTS

DIRECTIONS

Notes

RECIPE:

INGREDIENTS

DIRECTIONS

Notes

RECIPE:

INGREDIENTS

DIRECTIONS

Notes

RECIPE:

INGREDIENTS

DIRECTIONS

Notes

RECIPE:

INGREDIENTS

DIRECTIONS

Notes

RECIPE:

INGREDIENTS

DIRECTIONS

Notes

RECIPE:

INGREDIENTS

DIRECTIONS

Notes

RECIPE:

INGREDIENTS

DIRECTIONS

Notes

RECIPE:

INGREDIENTS

DIRECTIONS

Notes

RECIPE:

INGREDIENTS

DIRECTIONS

Notes

RECIPE:

INGREDIENTS

DIRECTIONS

Notes

RECIPE:

INGREDIENTS

DIRECTIONS

Notes

RECIPE:

INGREDIENTS

DIRECTIONS

Notes

RECIPE:

INGREDIENTS

DIRECTIONS

Notes

RECIPE:

INGREDIENTS

DIRECTIONS

Notes

RECIPE:

INGREDIENTS

DIRECTIONS

Notes

RECIPE:

INGREDIENTS

DIRECTIONS

Notes

RECIPE:

INGREDIENTS

DIRECTIONS

Notes

RECIPE:

INGREDIENTS

DIRECTIONS

Notes

RECIPE:

INGREDIENTS

DIRECTIONS

Notes

RECIPE:

INGREDIENTS

DIRECTIONS

Notes

RECIPE:

INGREDIENTS

DIRECTIONS

Notes

RECIPE:

INGREDIENTS

DIRECTIONS

Notes

RECIPE:

INGREDIENTS

DIRECTIONS

Notes

RECIPE:

INGREDIENTS

DIRECTIONS

Notes

RECIPE:

INGREDIENTS

DIRECTIONS

Notes

RECIPE:

INGREDIENTS

DIRECTIONS

Notes

RECIPE:

INGREDIENTS

DIRECTIONS

Notes

RECIPE:

INGREDIENTS

DIRECTIONS

Notes

RECIPE:

INGREDIENTS

DIRECTIONS

Notes

RECIPE:

INGREDIENTS

DIRECTIONS

Notes

RECIPE:

INGREDIENTS

DIRECTIONS

Notes

RECIPE:

INGREDIENTS

DIRECTIONS

Notes

RECIPE:

INGREDIENTS

DIRECTIONS

Notes

RECIPE:

INGREDIENTS

DIRECTIONS

Notes

RECIPE:

INGREDIENTS

DIRECTIONS

Notes

RECIPE:

INGREDIENTS

DIRECTIONS

Notes

RECIPE:

INGREDIENTS

DIRECTIONS

Notes

RECIPE:

INGREDIENTS

DIRECTIONS

Notes

RECIPE:

INGREDIENTS

DIRECTIONS

Notes

RECIPE:

INGREDIENTS

DIRECTIONS

Notes

RECIPE:

INGREDIENTS

DIRECTIONS

Notes

RECIPE:

INGREDIENTS

DIRECTIONS

Notes

RECIPE:

INGREDIENTS

DIRECTIONS

Notes

RECIPE:

INGREDIENTS

DIRECTIONS

Notes

RECIPE:

INGREDIENTS

DIRECTIONS

Notes

RECIPE:

INGREDIENTS

DIRECTIONS

Notes

RECIPE:

INGREDIENTS

DIRECTIONS

Notes

RECIPE:

INGREDIENTS

DIRECTIONS

Notes

RECIPE:

INGREDIENTS

DIRECTIONS

Notes

RECIPE:

INGREDIENTS

DIRECTIONS

Notes

RECIPE:

INGREDIENTS

DIRECTIONS

Notes

RECIPE:

INGREDIENTS

DIRECTIONS

Notes

RECIPE:

INGREDIENTS

DIRECTIONS

Notes

RECIPE:

INGREDIENTS

DIRECTIONS

Notes

RECIPE:

INGREDIENTS

DIRECTIONS

Notes

RECIPE:

INGREDIENTS

DIRECTIONS

Notes

RECIPE:

INGREDIENTS

DIRECTIONS

Notes

RECIPE:

INGREDIENTS

DIRECTIONS

Notes

RECIPE:

INGREDIENTS

Notes

DIRECTIONS

RECIPE:

INGREDIENTS

DIRECTIONS

Notes

RECIPE:

INGREDIENTS

DIRECTIONS

Notes

RECIPE:

INGREDIENTS

DIRECTIONS

Notes

RECIPE:

INGREDIENTS

DIRECTIONS

Notes

RECIPE:

INGREDIENTS

DIRECTIONS

Notes

RECIPE:

INGREDIENTS

DIRECTIONS

Notes

RECIPE:

INGREDIENTS

DIRECTIONS

Notes

RECIPE:

INGREDIENTS

DIRECTIONS

Notes

RECIPE:

INGREDIENTS

DIRECTIONS

Notes

RECIPE:

INGREDIENTS

DIRECTIONS

Notes

RECIPE:

INGREDIENTS

DIRECTIONS

Notes

RECIPE:

INGREDIENTS

DIRECTIONS

Notes

Made in the USA
Monee, IL
05 November 2026

67374715R00063